# Treating Her Own Immune System To Fight Cancer

# Treating Her Own Immune System To Fight Cancer

JBell Jones

To order additional copies of this book, contact:
Xlibris Corporation
1-888-795-4274
www.Xlibris.com
Orders@Xlibris.com
39105

Hello, Diary,

I have been going down health wise for sometime. It's 1996, and we are still looking for a health care provider to help me with these tumors in my abdomen and in the left side. I can feel them moving, and sometimes they leak into my bloodstream and sting. I am trying to find a female health care provider to help me. I know the tumor was there when the health care provider did my breast surgery in 1995, but they have started to leak into my system now. When I get sick, I feel the fluid leaking down my left leg. It usually happens when I have done some strenuous walking.


Hello, Diary,

I call a health care provider today, and I have an appointment with her office this month, September 1997.


Hello, Diary,

Nineteen ninety-seven, I went to my appointment today with the health care provider, I gave her my records from my last health care provider, and she ordered some test. She's nice and friendly.


Hello, Diary,

Nineteen ninety-seven, My health care provider's nurse called today; she said the test was fine. That's what the last health care provider told me a few weeks ago. She gave me an appointment for a mammogram next month. She did not give me any reason for the pain and stinging in my left side and back.

Hello, Diary,

December 1997. I went to the mall today with my sisters, which meant some walking and looking. Tonight, my body is stinging all over; even my eyes are stinging this time. I know something is going wrong in my body. I think the cancer has spread from my abdomen to other parts of my body; maybe it's the breast cancer spreading. I am disappointed again; no one cares or listens to us when we talk, and I do not think the tests are picking up the cancer; something is wrong with my body.

Hello, Diary,

February 1998. I had a sickle-cell crisis last night; the health care provider said I had an infection. She did not say where the infection was or what cause it. She gave me some Medication. My blood count was low as usual. I need a CT scan or a bone scan. It is hard when you have to ask for tests. Especially, when they think you are crazy anyway. Crazy is in my records. It's all in her mind, except for the pain in the left side of my body.

Hello, Diary,

February 17, 1998. I went for my sixth month appointment today. My health care provider says everything is the same. I feel a change taking in my body; it is frightening me. Something is wrong. I need to take my medical records to a health care provider in another state, and try to find someone to help me. I am sick and dying. When Earl gets out of the hospital, I will look in another state for medical help.

Hello, Diary,

August 20, 1998, another sixth month exam, I had my mammogram today. The nurse said my lump that was there on the last exam has moved; it disappeared. My body is still stinging, my stomach, ribs, and leg. I do not know what is going on in my body, but I am not crazy; something is wrong with my body.

Hello, Diary,

It's February 1999, and I still do not have an answer to the pain and stinging in my body. The health care providers keep saying there is nothing there showing up on the scans in my side, but they have seen something on my kidney, an ovary in the pass, that may be causing the problem. My body is aching all over; even behind my eyes is aching. I have blue knots coming under my skin on my legs and arms. I believe the cancer is spreading. My head, ribs, legs, and stomach are stinging more lately. I believe it has something to do with what is going on in my left side.

Hello, Diary,

July 1999. I have been in the hospital again since we last visited. I need to see a health care provider now, but I am so disappointed they think I am crazy. My ribs are stinging, my lower body is numb, and something is happening to my circulation. My foot is numb and sore all under the bottom. I do not want any more pain pills. Is there any way to treat black cancer?

Hello, Diary,

May 2000. I was so sick this weekend. I was out of town at my sister's house, so I suffered until Monday. I was feeling better on Monday; my sister encouraged me to get seen by a health care provider at the cancer center. The health care provider did some scans and sent me to see a kidney health care provider. He did some scans on my kidneys. I never could get him to talk to me about the test, so I wrote him for the results, and I received them through the mail. It said I had some nodes on my kidney on the left side. They were there back in 1995 when UK did the same test. The test will be paid for, which I did not receive the benefit from. I feel cheated again.

Hello, Diary,

It's October 9, 2000. I need some serious help with this cancer in my left back and abdomen. My left side stays cool; it's killing me, I have been drinking hot liquids to keep it warm. I thought my health care provider would be able to find the problem since she is a woman too. They said back in 1995 that no one was going to do anything about the pain in my left side, so for that, he has been right. I was hoping that a female health care provider would be different; women should try to listen to each other.

Hello, Diary,

October 23, 2000. Today I took my scan to a different health care provider. He said that he could not see anything usual, but my spleen was enlarged. The health care providers told me last year that my spleen is not there any longer; my sickle-cell disease had destroyed it. I saw the knot on the film he showed me. I wonder, is this what is affecting my back? He is sending me to a urologist for my kidney.

Hello, Diary,

October 2000. I had my appointment with the urologist. It was after 4:00 p.m., he must have had a long day because he slept all through my appointment; the minute he sat down, he went to sleep. He woke up and asked another question and went back to sleep again. I was not going to take any medicine if he had given me any, but he did not. So I left that office with a sick feeling in the pit of my stomach again. As specialist, did he read my films? I feel cheated again.

Hello, Diary,

It's November 3, 2000. My lab test came back with infection in my stomach again. The health care provider said he cannot treat me for the infection since I was treated back in February with medication. He told me to go back to the last health care provider for more follow-up. I feel so bad, and there is no answer for the feeling bad according to the medical professions.

Hello, Diary,

November 17, 2000. I went back to the gastroenterologist. She said she could not treat me again at this time; she was not going to do any more tests now. To come back in a month. She gave me something for acid reflux. I do not have the money to keep going to these appointments. I am driving myself half-sick, and the appointments take a long time in waiting to see the health care provider; I am sick.

Hello, Diary,

May 27, 2001. I awaken hurting in my stomach and back and vomiting; my left side was numb and stinging. The health care providers say they cannot find anything wrong; in the meantime, I am dying. Black cancer is always diagnosed as a mind problem, arthritis, or your other disease, until it is too late. I know my body, and this is a different kind of pain and stinging in my body. I am having problems walking and standing now. I am up most nights; my pain is so bad, and my body is sweating profusely because of the pain from the tumors in my abdomen. The tumors should have been removed back in 1995.

Hello, Diary,

June 1, 2001. I finally made an appointment with a health care provider out of state. He is a gastroenterologist. He took my medical history and drew some blood for testing. He said he would contact my health care provider back home, my lady health care provider. Since I was taking some medicine, he told me to continue to take it, and he would see me back in two weeks.

Hello, Diary,

June 15, 2001. I am back; this is my second appointment with the gastroenterologist. He gave me a quick look over my report in five minutes. He said nothing had change; he wrote me a prescription for Depression Medication. How does a gastroenterologist know that I need Depression Medication after just one visit? It's just arthritis or your nerve until the cancer has become so bad that it cannot be treated. I see why we are dying so often; cancer must be hard to find, and we are given Depression Medication or pain pills to cover the symptoms. Do you think all my travel and borrowing money was a waste?

Hello, Diary,

October 2001. I sent a letter to a popular talk show today.

Hello, Diary,

November 2001. I went to the cancer center in Blackstone today to try to talk to someone that might know what type of help I need. I still have not received an answer for the cause of the pain in my body, the abdomen, my head is stinging, my ribs is too and I am getting worse, the pain is getting hard to live with. The counsel subjected that I find a Internal Medicine health care provider to look at my stomach. So my friend and I set out to find a health care provider at once. I have been to some of the top health care providers; they are not hearing me. Something is going wrong in my body; there is too much pain. I am going to try a Internal Medicine doctor.

Hello, Diary,

November 20, 2001. I found a health care provider. She did some scan and a blood test. She said my blood iron level was low, so she called in a prescription to my drugstore. She is a medical student at the hospital where I had my breast surgery back in 1995.

Hello, Diary,

December 2001. I have not been able to get in touch with my interns yet; she was going to have some more tests done. My body is going down. I am trying to do what I can to help myself. I bought some ginger root to make some tea to drink to try to help my left side from staying so cool; it has helped.

Hello, Diary,

It's December 23, 2001. I had an appointment in TIN, with a health care provider today. She was so nice too. She said she was going to try to help me get an answer to my pain. She did not take state insurance, so my family had to pay her for this office visit. She set up a stomach x-ray and ultrasound for December 24.

Hello, Diary,

December 24, 2001. Today, I went to the TIN Hospital and had the test. That evening, my sister, brothers, and I went back over to the health care provider's office as she asked. The door of the office was open, but no one came to the desk. So we went back home. I will have to call back for the results.

Hello, Diary,

January 4, 2002. I called the TIN health care provider's office today to get the results of my test. The receptionist was very rude to me; she said that the health care provider had thirty reports, so she will get to me when she could. She would call me, that is not what she said three weeks ago; I was to get the report that same day. They were nice before I became a patient.

Hello, Diary,

It's February 8, 2002. I finally received a call from my TIN health care provider just five minutes before five o'clock. She said my blood was low and my bowel needed to be tested further in the future. When I met her, she said she was going to help me find the answer to my pain in my stomach; now it's back to me to go find someone.

Hello, Diary,

February 2002. I had my appointment with my health care provider; she said everything is fine. I told her about the stinging in my head and ribs again. There was only a look; there was someone with her today, I thought it was a new health care provider, but she is a drug rep. No relief for me this time.

Hello, Diary,

It's May 18, 2002. Tomorrow, I am having an endoscopy at UK. Everything is stinging, and something feels like it's being released into my bloodstream on the left side of my body. I do not believe the test can find out what is in my side unless they operate. The test kept coming back fine, but I am sick and in pain.

Hello, Diary,

September 23, 2002. My health care provider called me yesterday. She said she needed to talk with me about the CT scan of my back, stomach, and head.

September 27, 2002. Today, I went to see my health care provider; she told me the scan shows what look like bone cancer. There were spots on my skull, ribs, and pelvis. So this pain and stinging that is going on in body is not just in my mind; I am not crazy. I had a chest x-ray in August that showed everything was looking good. The health care provider asked if I was still able to hold my bowel and bladder since the cancer is on my spine too. I said yes, but there is stinging and numbness in the area. The health care provider examined me from top to bottom for tumors. I am up most nights in pain and having difficulty in walking. Today, I thank Jar that a friend was with me at the time; it made the bad news easer to receive. I thank her too for offering to take me to the health care provider today. Now I have to tell my family. I know they will be okay. I really hate to tell my brother who is paralyzed that I may soon be paralyzed from cancer on my spine. I am the only one who is not working at this time, so I can check on him often.

Hello, Diary,

September 27, 2002. I will tell my sisters and brothers today. I hate to do it, but I am going to need their help getting a second opinion soon. Earl and Tonne came by first. I told them and they were very encouraging to me. Earl told me to try to stay strong and fight the disease. He is a good example, since his accident in 1998, in which he broke his neck and injured his spine leaving him paralyzed. He has always been a fighter. I told W. C., and he told Jr. Lee, and her daughter came over, so I told them about my health. They said they would help all they can so I can get a second opinion. Later, I called Dean and Chris; they were very encouraging too. They offered to help me in any way they could. They have been going with me out of state trying to get an answer to the pain in my side and stomach. I thank you all; I want to live, even though I am forty something with sickle-cell. I have an appointment with a cancer health care provider in TIN on Tuesday at the cancer center.

Hello, Diary,

October 2002. Today starts a new chapter in my life, a few more years of trying to battle this cancer. The health care provider at the cancer center said if the cancer is in my bones, I will probably have two years; he seems to be a good health care provider. I think this cancer center is part of a group of cancer centers. I was very surprise at my reaction. I did not cry this time. I felt that God held me up today. The health care provider said that until we know the source of the cancer, he cannot be sure of the number of years; it could be more or less. I believe it is ovarian or kidney cancer. My left side and stomach have been hurting and stinging for years it has spread all over. I have been receiving a checkup every six months and have been seen by at lease five health care providers in the past few years who are experts in their fields, but they just do not listen.

Hello, Diary,

It's October 8, 2002. Chris and I started out on the evening of October 7 for my sister's house to spend the night so we could get an early start tomorrow for TIN. My appointment is at 8:00 a.m. tomorrow. I tried to keep a positive outlook, but I know the situation is serious. We made it to the cancer center on time the next day. The health care provider saw me on time; he said he did not see any brain or chest cancer. He said there was some bone lesion on my bone scans. He stated to recommend hormones treatment, but decided to bring me back for a PET scan. He asked me to bring all of my other CT scans and x-rays from the past. He said UK had sent him my breast cancer sample, and it was receptor positive cancer. I do not understand this. I know something is wrong in my body, with all this stinging and pain in my head, ribs, and bones. I am having trouble in walking now. We left the cancer center hopeful. My family and friends have been really helpful to me. My best friend gave me a tape last month on vitamins and minerals from a health care provider that had done some studies on the immune system. So I am starting this and a special diet I was told about this month.

Hello, Diary,

October 14, 2002. I started the vitamins, minerals, and vegetable diet today. My friends have been trying to give me all the helpful tips they can until I get a second opinion on the cancer. So I am trying everything. I am eating different and am on the vitamin and mineral program. Each day I get my handful of vitamins and my ounces of liquids as I start my day. This goes on three times a day.—

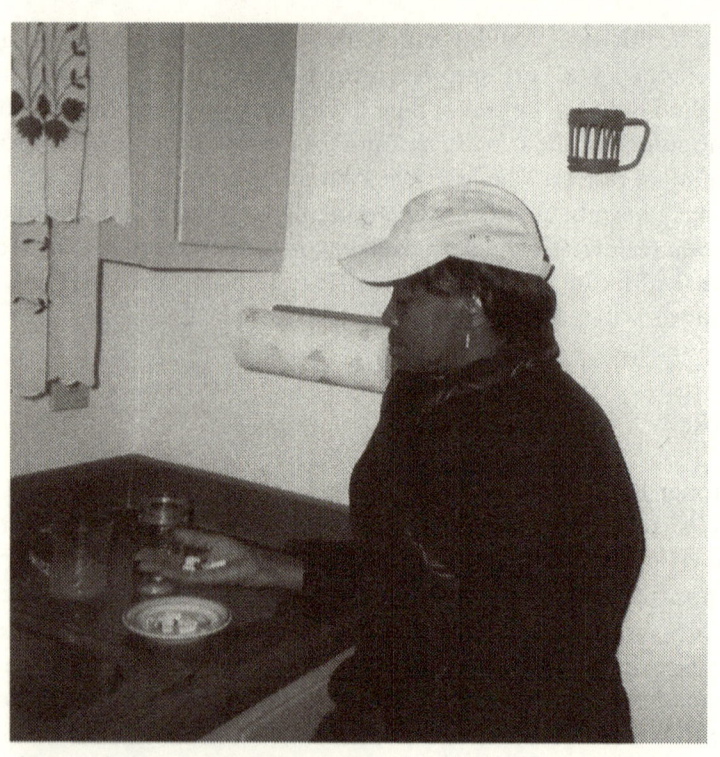

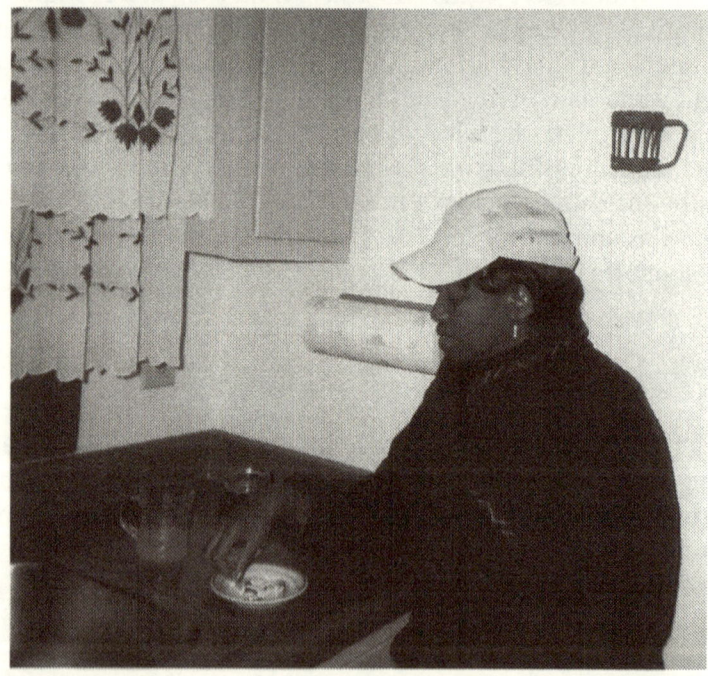

Hello, Diary,

Jr. Lee and I left Yat City at 4:00 a.m. for TIN because I had to have the PET scan at 7:00 a.m. I am taking my scan from G. W. I will have to travel back to TIN next week to get my results.

Hello, Diary,

October 22, 2002. I have an appointment at 12:00 noon at the cancer center in TIN. Chris, Lee, and I left Yat City at 9:00 a.m. I was finally to get an answer from all these tests today, a yes or no answer. The health care provider came in the room; he gave me the results. To my surprise, he said he was not sure what was on the scan from UK, but the PET scan did not show any cancer. There was something on the scan from UK. The health care provider said it did not look like anything serious. I asked about the stinging in my ribs, stomach, and head. He did not have an answer. "What about some treatment?" I asked. He said he could not suggested anything until he could take a look at the scans in the year 2000 from the other hospitals. I gave the films to the radiologist last Tuesday, as he had asked me to do, for him to read and send him the report along with the PET scan. He was supposed to have them today. I drove fifty miles on Friday to get the films from UK and another fifty miles on Monday to G. W. to get the other films, so I could give them to his radiologist last Tuesday, and now they did not read the films. I used ALL of my little energy, time, and money for nothing. I will have to come back to TIN again. Someone is not being professional, or they just do not care, it not them. So we went home not knowing the answer again. I was so discouraged that when we stopped to eat, I went off my diet. I should have had a salad, but I ate a meal.

Hello, Diary,

November 3, 2002. I had a assembly day today in Green Town. I return home about 7:00 p.m. I am sick; it is a cool day today. I warmed up and started hurting, so I took some pain medicine. At 12:00 noon, I was completely sick. I called my sister to come and take me to the hospital. The health care provider said my sickle-cell was in crisis because my blood was so low. I needed blood, but I do not take blood for personal reasons. He gave me a pain shot and some drip in my veins. The health care provider wanted to admit me the hospital. I asked to go to UK because they were testing to see if the cancer had return. Bertha and I left there for UK at 2 p.m. that night. I was in pain from my waist down. The health care provider at UK said I needed blood too, but I do not take blood. He gave me m-short and sent me home at 8:00 a.m. On Tuesday, I had an appointment with my health care provider at UK Clinic, so I was in bed all day Monday in pain. Tuesday, my friend took me to my appointment at 2:00 p.m. When the health care provider checked, my temperature was 100.2. I was having chills, so she admitted me to UK and ordered me a short and a drip. The next morning, the pain was almost gone, so I was told that I had an infection, but they could not find out where it was from. I was sent home. I was feeling better until next time; there is always a next time for us sickle-cell patients, I have had three infections this year alone. What's causing them? What's going on in my left side? My kidney? After eight months, I still do not know if I have cancer that has spread to my bone. I have had so many health care providers since 1995. This pain in my abdomen and left side is affecting my whole body now.

Hello, Diary,

November 21, 2002. I called the cancer health care provider in TIN. Today the nurse gave me an appointment for November 26. I still do not have a true diagnosis yet. It's like I am in mid-air. I am taking the vitamins and minerals, and they are doing more for me than anything so far in helping me. If I were not on them, I would be dead now. I think vitamins would work even better if I had some medicine along with the supplement.

Hello, Diary,

November 26, 2002. I went to my appointment at the cancer center in TIN. The health care provider said he did not see any bone cancer, but they could not see the full picture from the CT scans from UK and GW. So he is going to have an abdomen and pelvis contrast scan done on December 3, 2002. He said the other scans were clouded. I have been dealing with this bone pain since the year 2000. I think cancer kills you not all at once, but it slowly eats away at you. It is really cold in TIN. I am sick today; my leg is numb on the left side. The blood is not flowing well on that side of my body. I still do not have a sure medical answer about my health, or any medical treatment.

Hello, Diary,

December 3, 2002. I had the abdomen and pelvis scan today in TIN. It's cold; my friend and her daughter went with me this time. The trip took all day; we are tired out. It was 7:00 p.m. tonight when we made it home; both of them have colds. I do not have the money to keep up these trips to TIN; it is going to stop, even if I do not get any answer to my health problem.

Hello, Diary,

December 10, 2002. My sister and I left her at 5:00 a.m. for TIN. Today I am to get the results of last week's scans. The appointment is at 9:00 a.m. We made it to TIN at 8:00 a.m. so we stopped to eat breakfast. At the health care provider's office at 9:00 a.m., the nurse put us into a room; the health care provider came in with the results. He found the same markings on the scans, but they have not changed in the last months from September to December. He did not think it is cancer but the effects of my sickle-cell damage. I asked why; the pain and stinging in my bones and body. He did not have an answer for it, but he saw two nodes on my kidney pole. He said I need to have a biopsy of the node. It was there in 2000 when the GW did the scan. The health care provider said it was not anything to worry about; everyone has them. I am still in the same situation I was in when I started months ago. Is it cancer that has spread to my ribs, skull, spine, and pelvis? No medical answer while the cancer spread through my body. I will have to come back for more tests.

Hello, Diary,

December 2002. I am sick today. I could not get an appointment until February 18, 2003. I am treating my own cancer with the juice, vitamins, and minerals to keep from dying.

Hello, Diary,

December 21, 2002. I have lost twenty-five pounds since October. Along with my supplement, I was instructed to stay off the sweets, fried food, and soft drink. The supplement will strengthen my immune system to fight the cancer. My ribs, skull, and pelvis are not stinging as bad as they were back months ago. I can walk better without so much pain. I have been treated like a hot potato, passed back and forward to the health care providers with a handful of reports. I have come to believe that cancer is not easy to diagnose with the scans; I know there is some cancer in my left abdomen and body. My body is hurting and stinging for a reason. The vitamins and minerals have helped, so I will keep taking them.

Hello, Diary,

December 26, 2002. I went with a friend to the funeral home to view the body of her cousin who died as a result of cancer. She is younger than I am, under fifty. It is another black cancer case. She probably went to the health care provider for years complaining, but it fell on deaf ears too. When she was treated, it was too little, too late; the cancer had spread everywhere. We are not taken seriously. We are given some pain pills or mind pills, until it is too late for treatment to work. She is so pretty. Our infected organs are not taking out until cancer spread to other organs. I look at her lying there so still and cold, knowing if it was not for God, my family, and friends, I would have been in her same situation some time ago. There are so many black women in our area dying of cancer, young women. I have been suffering for years, trying to get help for what is going on in my left side, the tumors that needs removing. Everything is being affected in my abdomen.

Hello, Diary,

December 30, 2002. I called a foundation. I talked to one of the members in an overseeing position there. He was not a health care provider, but he told me that they were working with the same vitamin provider that I was getting vitamins and minerals from the last three months. I told him that my friend had given me the health care provider's tape to listen to, and I was feeling some better now. I told him I was trying to stay on the supplement because I do believe the health care provider when she said it is cancer on my spine, ribs, and skull. It feels different from the sickle-cell pain in the left side of my body. The foundation could not help me with any health needs other than give me some suggestion.

Hello, Diary,

January 21, 2003. I was at the clinic for my appointment today. The health care provider told me to stop taking my iron pills because they can damage my heart. He gave me some appointments for test, bone scan, and ultrasound. I had the reports from my TIN health care provider, but he told me to keep the report. Money down the drain, health care providers paid me (patient) nothing, waiting some more months. It's necessary for me to keep treating my own immune system to strengthen my system to fight my cancer

Hello, Diary,

February 16, 2003. Good morning, black cancer, arthritis, or sickle cell; my right arm has a large blue knot on it, and my abdomen is stinging again today. A friend gave me a number to a health care provider in Moon Town; he said this health care provider would give me an answer in a week. It is different for me. It's not the same; we want it to be the same treatment for all. I would like to move outer state, but I have other responsibilities.

Hello, Diary,

March 4, 2003. A infection in my body brought me to the hospital this morning. I keep getting these infections. I think it is because of the tumors in my abdomen. The emergency room health care provider said I have a high white blood count. The only thing he could do is to treat me for the pain. This has been an agitating week; a family member is in the hospital with a problem with their heart, and their daughter just had surgery. Who is going to take care of all of us sick people? We are living in times hard to deal with; there is so much going on in our lives. Sometimes all the problems make it hard to see your way out of this mess.

Hello, Diary,

March 19, 2003. I am tired out today. I had an appointment at the clinic. I was to get results of my test on my heart, bones, and kidney. The health care provider said it looks as my heart vale is flowing backward. Is that possible? There is something on my kidney, and it could be cancer on my spine, but he was not sure. I need another CT scan, so more test in the next few weeks. It's getting hard to deal.

At 2:00 p.m. I had an appointment with the health care provider. I asked her about my tests. She said my heart was okay. It was different from what the health care provider had said an hour ago. She said my bone scan showed that there was something on my spine, ribs, and skull. It could be sickle cell, or it could be cancer. I asked what if it is cancer. She said we will keep watching it. I have been begging my cancer health care provider the last two years to help me because my ribs and skull had been stinging so bad. The health care provider gave me some pain pills and some Depression Medication. The health care provider gave me an appointment for an EKG. What am I to do? I am physically, emotionally, and financially exhausted.

Hello, Diary,

March 24, 2003. The health care provider's nurse in TIN called today. She said I had an appointment with the health care provider tomorrow. I am going to ask my brother to miss his college classes and work to take me to TIN tomorrow. The last few times my younger brother had miss work to take me to the TIN appointments. The traveling is too expensive. I am financially broke and using credit to make these trips.

Hello, Diary,

March 25, 2003. To TIN again. I met my brother at a truck stop at 7:00 p.m. of the interstate to save time. My brother had worked all night, so I drove to TIN. I felt so bad he had to make that sacrifice to go with me, but I thank them all. It will take the whole day, and he has to work again tonight. It's three hundred miles one way. We made it to the appointment. The health care provider at first said he could not help me anymore. He had not helped me yet to get an answer. He only worked with patients who had already been diagnosed with cancer in certain parts of their body. He did not say that when he first saw me as a patient. I came to him for a second opinion, to get him to pinpoint where the cancer was. So I started crying, because I cannot take any more uncertainty. All of them, he and those back home, are hiding something. I told him I was not going back to UK. He said he would take a look at my scans again. Come back in a week.

Hello, Diary,

March 31, 2003. My sister and I started for TIN at 6:00 a.m. today. I saw the health care provider at 11:00 a.m. He did not see anything different; he believes it is damaged sickle-cell on my ribs, skull, and spine. He asked, "What did my cancer health care provider say back home?" I wanted to say if she knew, I would not have been in his office today. I have been pledging with her for almost two years to help me with this pain in my ribs and skull. He gave me an appointment for another scan on Friday. My heart is figuratively bleeding. I will just double up on my supplement, treating my own immune system to fight the cancer.

Hello, Diary,

April 8, 2003. Back to TIN, to the health care provider's office to get the result of this CT scan. The health care provider said my bones and kidney markings have not changed over the past months. He did not have any answer to the pain and stinging in my body. He said he could not do anything further for me; he suggested that I get a breast exam soon. I will have to keep trying to treat myself with the supplement. We came home like we started out six months ago, and with thousands of dollars spent.

Hello, Diary,

April 9, 2003. Today, I wrote the insurance office to try to get help with buying my vitamins and minerals. I asked them for some financial assistance to help buy supplement to help fight my cancer. So I have been treating my own immune system since October 2002.

Hello, Diary,

April 12, 2003. I receive a letter from the insurance office saying that my request for help has been forwarded to their office of beneficiary relation division in Blackstone, who will be able to give me an answer.

Hello, Diary,

April 16, 2003. I called the cancer treatment center today. After getting my information from the personnel, the person said that they did not take State insurance. They can't take me as a patient unless I deposit $25,000 in a bank account. She, said she hopes I can get some help at another clinic. I needed these tumors in my abdomen removed five years ago. Now this cancer has spread everywhere in my body.

Hello, Diary,

April 22, 2003. Today, I was told that most health care providers think we sickle-cell patients just want pain pills. I told them I realized that may be true with some patients and health care providers, but not everyone is looking for drugs;I am not, but pain medicine is what we get. I have a serious problem that had been neglected. I need someone to help me get the help I need. I thank her for your information. I already knew that was true.

Hello, Diary,

April 30, 2003. Today, an oncology nurse from the cancer society called me back because I had asked for help. She said the only thing she could do is to tell me to go to a pain management health care provider. I ask, "Can they help with vitamin supplements for cancer patients?" She said no, they did not offer that kind of help.

Hello, Diary,

May 1, 2003. I have been feeling so bad lately, so I decided to go to the downtown clinic. When the nurse checked me in, she said I had used all of my twelve health care providers on my State Insurance for the year. I did not have the $72 for the visit today. I have an appointment with my health care provider on May 20. I have read somewhere that HP will help infections. My left side was infected, so I went home and took a little hydrogen peroxide for the infection. Between the sickle cell and the cancer, I use up my twelve health care provider visits before the year is out.

Hello, Diary,

May 8, 2003. My best friend called today. She ordered me some vitamins and minerals. I am thankful that she introduced me to the supplement back in October 2002. I, most likely, would be dead by now, but they have helped me to keep going, and my bones have improved some. The ribs, skull, and spine are not stinging as bad as they were, and they feel stronger now. I will go to her house tomorrow and get the vitamins. Stand by, cancer.

Hello, Diary,

May 13, 2003. My cousin from Illinois gave me a number to the Quart Clinic to try to get checked by them. He had his cancer treated at that clinic. So I called today. I talked to the person for appointments; she took my information then connected me to a person in the financial department. That person said the Quart Clinic did not take State Insurance patients. She said that to get seen, I need an up-front deposit of $3,300 at the clinic. So my heart sunk again. She said there were too many people like me, with needs but no insurance, which is true. I have been to all the cancer organizations to ask for help, but there is none for us. So I am No.********* on the Book.

Hello, Diary,

May 20, 2003. I went to my appointment with my health care provider today. She did some blood tests; she said they looked okay. She will be graduating in July, so I will get another student health care provider next time and have to start all over again. I came home empty. So I will have to keep treating myself with my vitamins and minerals to help with the cancer.

Hello, Diary,

July 2, 2003. Today, I talked to a local newspaper reporter to try to get a grant to go to the Quart Clinic. I prayed that the article is not too much an embarrassment to my family or would not cause me any problems. The reporter was very nice, so I hope I can find some help.

Hello, Diary,

July 25, 2003, Tuesday, I went to Glenda to make an appointment with a health care provider that a friend told me was his health care provider, and the health care provider is a very good cancer health care provider. I have an appointment for August 12, 2003. I am feeling like a wet dog today. I am feeling infected again. I am going to take some more HP. It seems like it is helping. I feel better after a few days of taking it.

Hello, Diary,

August 8, 2003. This evening, all of my problems had just become too much for me: the bills, the medicine, the cards, and no cash in hand. I have begged so much that there is no one left to beg. My family and friends has helped to the limit; all I could do is sit on the floor and cry and pray to Jar. I asked, a Community Organization for help with light bills, but they said no, they would not help me. My vitamins and minerals were out. I cannot go without them, without being in severe pain. As I was crying, my mind recalled something that was said to a Bible student this week: Trust in God! My mind, heart, and tears stopped racing. That same evening, a classmate and friend from high school called and said she and some other classmates had read my article in the newspaper. They had cards for me; and she and her husband would bring it to me tomorrow. It was like God said, "Just trust me." I could only cry again, but with thankfulness.

Hello, Diary,

September 12, 2003. I had my first MRI at the new health care provider's office on my spine and other x-rays. It has been a whole year now, and I still do not know how far the cancer has spread in my body. Did I have breast cancer or not? In ninety-five, something is not right with the answers I am receiving from the medical experts. Could it have been a cancer in another part of my body in the first place? I do not have the money to keep up this traveling. Today is going to be a long day. I do not know how we are going to do it. I am at one end of the state, and a family is at the other end having surgery to remove a large tumor from behind her heart. So I will drive back to my sister's home, and we will drive another 120 miles at 5:00 p.m. this evening to see her. Our family is under so much stress now. The girls have been sick this last year.

Hello, Diary,

September 13, 2003. The family member came through the surgery, but they is in bad shape. The surgery was very extensive, back, ribs and chest all cut. I feel so sorry for them. The tumor has been there for sometime. We are thankful that they survived. It will be a long recovery for them.

Hello, Diary,

September 23, 2003. I am up at 6:00 a.m. this morning to drive to Glenda for my appointment at 9:00 a.m. I am nervous about what I am going to hear this time, praying not to break down. The health care provider came in the examination room. He asked me how I was today and how old I was. I told him. He said I have a tumor close to my spine, but he could not remove it. He said he would start treating me today. He was going to treat me with two medicines; one was a pill and one was a drip in the veins. Finally, someone heard me and was going to do something to treat me. I thanked him, and my friend that told me about the health care provider who is very good. We talked, and I received my prescription and appointment. I received the drip today, and I will start my pills tomorrow.

Hello, Diary,

September 24, 2003. I took my pill today at 5:00 p.m., and it is 8 p.m., and I am having chills. I am going from chills to fever at 1:00 p.m. I am weak and sweating. I must be having side effects from the pills.

Hello, Diary,

September 28, 2003. Today I have a rash under my left foot and my right hand. It is burning and swollen; the nerve in both of my hands is shot. When I touch anything, there is pain. I will stop taking the pills until I talk to the health care provider. I tried to keep taking it, but it's causing more nerve pain. The medicine must be killing something because my left foot is black, and the nerves in my hand are shot when I touch anything. I am going to ask the health care provider to take me of this medication and give me another medication.

Hello, Diary,

October 3, 2003. I was back at the health care provider's office at 8:00 a.m. My brother worked all night last night, but he took me to the health care provider this today. We talked to the nurse about the rash and swelling in my hand and feet. She said it were not from the drugs, but it only started after my treatment with these drugs. I asked her what stage my cancer was in; she did not know. My brother and I were back in Yat City at 1:00 p.m. He was so tired out. He headed for home about an hour away. After ten minutes, he was back at my door; his car's fan belt had broken. There was no shop in Yat City, so I had to drive him the hour away to look for the car part. He found the car part and was back in Yat City by 7:00 p.m., but the part would not fit the car. Just as we were trying to think what to do next, my younger brother drove up. He had a truck and trailer, so they put the car on the trailer and headed back home with my brother's car. He has been up twenty-four hours, and I am worried about his health now. Both of them are tired physically and mentally. On my next trip to the health care provider on October 24, I will be going alone. The only positive thing out of today is we spent some family time together.

Hello, Diary,

October 14, 2003. The lady from the University of X Cancer Trial Center called me back today to let me know that they did not have a clinical trial that would fit my case. It's hard to believe that there is not anything the clinic can do for my cancer. You hear about new clinic trials all the time.

Hello, Diary,

October 24, 2003. I was really sick this week, so I was not able to go get my drip today. I reschedule my appointment for next week. Some friends came over to bring me some fruit and juice, which is a blessing when you live alone and have to do almost everything for yourself, sick or not. It is really good to have someone to come by to see you. It will take your mind out of your pain for a minute, because there is so much going on with others too. I see I am not suffering alone.

Hello, Diary,

October 30, 2003. I am just going to have to take some more HP; my abdomen is infected again. Something has been going wrong in my abdomen a long time now. The tumors should have been removed back in 1995. I have been out of my good vitamins and minerals for some time now. They have been helping to keep me alive and going since 2002. Financially, I have a problem; it's so hard on a limited income when you are sick. I need to move closer to the health care provider's office, the gas, the driving, and my car; it's just too much.

Hello, Diary,

November 2003. I had to stop taking my pills because they were still causing my rash and feet to turn blue and were damaging the nerves in my right hand and wrist. I ask the nurse could I come in to get the health care provider to change my medicine. She told me to go to my family health care provider. I told her that I would stop taking the medicine. The health care provider will change the medicine on my next visit.

Hello, Diary,

November 6, 2003. The health care provider at Center Town had seen me today for my hands and feet. He gave me a prescription and told me to get some J. cream for my feet.

Hello, Diary,

November 13, 2003. The medicine did start clearing up the rash on my feet; the hand and wrist were better too. The cancer pills caused the bone in my hand and wrist to puff up, which is still there, but the nerve's sensation was getting better also. The vitamins and minerals were a wonder for me. I am so glad my friend gave me that health care provider tape back in 2002. They have spared me some pain too.

Hello, Diary,

November 19, 2003. I tried to get a cancer health care provider back in Blackstone to be closer than Glenda, but the health care providers wanted to put me back with my last cancer health care provider who, for two years, I begged to help me with the stinging in my ribs, head, and left side. They looked at me as crazy. I do not want to go back there again.

Hello, Diary,

December 23, 2003. My eyes have been red and stinging for a couple of weeks now, so I had them tested today. The health care provider said there was no problem with my eyes, so it's not coming from my skull; I just needed glasses.

Hello, Diary,

December 24, 2003. I received my Drediv drip today for my bones. I hope to be feeling much better soon now that I am getting the Drediv drip. I thank my health care provider for finding me the right drug to treatment my cancer. I have not had any side effects from this medication yet. I have seen the nurse for my wrist and hand; she gave me a prescription.

Hello, Diary,

January 3, 2004. I found out that one of my past neighbors and friends died last year from cancer. She is younger than I. She was at the clinic to see the health care providers as much as I was. How could the cancer be so advanced? Why is it that no one knows any signs of early cancer when we go for medical treatment? I had all the signs that were in the cancer book for breast cancer that had spread. When I received the book from the cancer society, my mouth fell open; those were the same symptoms I had been feeling for almost two years. Something is wrong with the testing, and the health care providers are not listening to us. We are told it is just arthritis, and we suffer from it until it is too late; the cancer kills us.

Hello, Diary,

January 26, 2004. Today, I went to Glenda to get the results of my CT scan. The health care provider said my head and chest were clear. He said the pain in my left side could be from my nerves coming from my spine. It feels like something is leaking in my side from time to time. The health care provider is going to check my blood for the next two weeks and order me an MRI in March.

Hello, Diary,

February 12, 2004. I went back to get my blood counts today. They were low, but they are always low. I will get them checked again on February 26.

Hello, Diary,

February 16, 2004. The spine is letting me know I have a problem today. The left side of my back and stomach is usually cold today. This cold spot has been in my side since 2000. I am off my vitamins and minerals this week, but the only thing, I can do is order the vitamins or wait and die. I need to keep treating my immune system to fight the cancer, to stay alive longer. It would be great if the medical community and cancer researcher do some clinical trails to study the effects of supplements on cancer patients. This would hopful open a opportunity to get supplements under insurance to treat cancer.

Hello, Diary,

February 26, 2004. I receive my blood count. It's the same. I was told something that was strange to me, that I have a mass on my kidney, but does it need treating? I asked about getting another round of chemotherapy because my left side and flesh were hurting. I was given a prescription. This may be all I need. I will keep treating my own immune system to fight the cancer with my vitamins and minerals.

Hello, Diary,

March 25, 2004. Today my body was stinging all over, but I had to drive myself to Glenda, the seventy miles to get my cancer treatment. It was God and me; the drive is getting to me, I need to move. I am thankful that I made it there and back home safe again.

Hello, Diary,

March 30, 2004. Judy went for a test today. Her children and we, two sisters, went with them. The test was long; the health care provider had found some polyps. He removed what he could and made an appointment with a surgeon to remove the rest of the polyps. We were all worried because cancer is in the family line. This means all three of the girls are ill. We left the health care provider's office trying to be positive. On the way home, we were in a major car accident. Judy and her daughter had to be taken back to the hospital. This possibly could have saved her life because she had no potassium in her system when the health care provider examined her. They went home that night, after a long day of suffering through surgery and the car accident.

Hello, Diary,

April 21, 2004. Judy had surgery today. The surgeon came out about ten o'clock and said it was going good. At eleven o'clock, the surgery was over, and she was in recovery. The surgeon said he looked around in the stomach and did not see any more tumors. She should be fine now. She will be in the hospital for a few days, and they will test her every year.

Hello, Diary,

April 27, 2004. Today, my other sister and I went to Glenda to get the results of my MRI and my Drediv drip. The health care provider said my spine had improved. It is the drip, pill, and all these high-price vitamins and minerals I am taking. As soon as I run out of my supplements, my pain is as it was in 2002. Since Judy was released from the hospital today, we stopped to see her. She was in some pain still. Her daughter has come home; she has been a great help to her. She is home with her for a month.

Hello, Diary,

May 25, 2004. I went to get my Drediv drip today. My blood count was very low. My body is doing its stinging thing today. The health care provider is sending me to Ford to get a PET scan on June 8. The scans always come back fine; they do not pick up cancer until it is too late.

Hello, Diary,

June 8, 2004. I went to Ford for my PET scan today.

Hello, Diary,

June 11, 2004. I awaken this morning vomiting, so I called the health care provider's office to talk with the nurse. She did not think I had an infection. She told me to get some over-the-counter medicine. I took some more HP to stop the bubbling in my stomach.


Hello, Diary,

July 20, 2004. I saw the health care provider and got my Drediv treatment today. The health care provider looked at my right hand that has been hurting. He said it is arthritis in my wrist.


Hello, Diary,

August 4, 2004. Dr. K had a bone scan done last week. He said the scan showed there was arthritis in my hand, wrist, shoulder, and thigh bones. Could it be where the cancer is affecting me?


Hello, Diary,

September 14, 2004. I was not feeling my best today, but I had to drive myself to get my Drediv treatment and exam. The health care provider said everything was the same. He did not need to change anything; my blood was low as usual, and I could get a shot once a week. I cannot afford the gas to drive the seventy miles four times a month, so I will try to build my blood by eating more vegetables and doubling my supplements.


Hello, Diary,

October 5, 2004. My system is infected. It seems like the fluid is leaking out of my abdomen down my left leg; my body is stinging. I am out of my good vitamins and minerals because I cannot afford them now. So I do not have anything in my body to fight the cancer; my immune system is weak. I need to improve my finances, so I can order the supplement.

Hello, Diary,

October 22, 2004. I had my visit with the health care provider today. She said the last CT scan showed that I had a mask on my kidney, so she ordered another CT scan on my kidney. I have been hurting for years in my side now.

Hello, Diary,

November 10, 2004. I am back on my good supplements today; I had my Drediv drip, and I am feeling pretty good.

Hello, Diary,

November 17, 2004. Today, my stomach and back are stinging again so bad. The problem is coming from the wall of my abdomen and intestines. I need a health care provider to look inside of my abdomen with a microscope. I will have to keep on taking my vitamins and minerals to keep fighting the cancer. People are tired of hearing me complain about my pain; they have their own problems. I just try to keep going and tell myself; I am okay. I could be doing worse.

Hello, Diary,

November 29, 2004. Today, I saw a news report on TV about a lady with advance cancer who was pleading to keep her marijuana as a medicine for her cancer. She touched a cord with me because I know without my vitamins and minerals, I would not be able to walk now. She said about two hours after taking the marijuana, she could walk on her own; her husband did not have to help her. When I tried to stop my vitamins and minerals, my body went back to its previous state of pain as it was before in 2002. My bones hurt so bad; I cannot move. My flesh is stinging; the cancer has spread across my body now. They say the test shows nothing wrong with my abdomen and left side, but I am in pain for some reason.

Hello, Diary,

December 14, 2004. I went to Glenda to get my Drediv drip today. The long drive is getting harder and harder to make. I am growing tired, and my car is wearing out too. We both are wearing out. The health care provider said everything was the same; my blood count was low, but it is always low. I need to be back closer to home for treatment. I cried most of the way home, I am just sick and tired from this long drive.

Hello, Diary,

January 12, 2005. My best friend, C. G. took off from her job today to take me to my appointment to get my Drediv in Glenda. We started out at 8:00 a.m. this morning and made it to Glenda at 9:00. After my treatment, she went to visit some friends in Glenda. After we ate lunch; C.G. drove another fifty miles to see a cousin. It was a small intermission to take my mind of things. We stayed a while and visited and ate cake with Lin. It was about six o'clock when we made it back to Yat City. C. had to drive another fifty miles home. We were bone tired, but I sure do thank C. Girl, for her kindness.

Hello, Diary,

January 14, 2005. I called an oncologist's office out of the Blackstone yellow pages today. The nurse said they could take me as a patient. I told her that I wanted to transfer from Glenda to Blackstone to be closer to home. She told me to have my records transferred to their office. So I called my health care provider's office and asked them to transfer the records, and they said they would. I gave the new health care provider's their name and telephone number. I am just worn out from the traveling.

Hello, Diary,

January 21, 2005. I was in Blackstone, picking up some vitamins today, so I picked up an application for apartment in Blackstone. If I get a health care provider in Blackstone, I am thinking about moving to be even closer the office, so I will not have to drive so much.

Hello, Diary,

February 9, 2005. My sister and I went to Glenda to get my Drediv drip today. The nurse said they were trying to transfer my medical records to that health care provider, but they were having a problem making the transformation to the Blackstone office.

Hello, Diary,

February 19, 2005. I found out that this health care provider uses the same oncologist services as the health care provider I left in 2002. I did not know this when I made the appointment, and the nurse did not know me at the time until they look at my information. So they would not take me as a patient. All the Blackstone oncologists work together, so I could not get one to take me as a patient.

Hello, Diary,

March 1, 2005, I went to a nonprofit meeting today. I am trying to learn how to start a nonprofit organization. I want to start a program to help patients with vitamins and minerals, especially those with breast cancer. We need help with buying supplements to build our immune system when fighting cancer. The meeting is a two-day meeting. There are so many regulations to learn, and you need to have finances up front to get started. I do not have the finances to get started, but I am going to try what they taught us in the meeting. My health is a major obstacle. There is no one that will hire someone with my health problems. It is hard to get help if you need it. If you do not need help, everyone is willing to give their time, energy, and finances. I don't know how long I can go on treating my immune system with these expensive supplements, but if I stop, I am going to die. I am trying to start a program to help me and others with cancer.

Hello, Diary,

March 12, 2005. Today, for the first time, my body started to do what the health care provider asked me about back in 2002. My spine must be relaxing. I have not had my Drediv or my good vitamins and minerals. I will ask the health care provider in Glenda if he can start giving me my Drediv again, and I double up on the vitamins.

Hello, Diary,

March 14, 2005. My brother is having knee surgery today. My sister, her daughter, and I went to be with him and his wife. The surgery went well. On the way home, I told my sister that I was going to ask my health care provider to take me back as a patient, so I can get my Drediv soon.

March 22, 2005. I receive my Drediv today. The other health care provider would not take me as his patient. He is associated with my former health care provider. My health care team here was nice to me as usual. They gave me my treatment, prescription, and did not say a thing. I am so thankful to them for their kindness in taking me back as a patient.

Hello, Diary,

April 8, 2005. The health care provider who was trying to help me to find a cancer health care provider closer to home, called today to tell me that he could not get a health care provider to take me as a patient. He said I should go back to my health care provider in Glenda. I told him I went back. I thanked him for his concern, but they took me back as a patient.

Hello, Diary,

May 2, 2005. My close friend, Alisha, died of breast cancer this morning. It was a shock to hear it. I know she was serious, but I did not think she would die this soon. We have been searching for help for four years now. If we had been treated early in the stages, things could have been different for us. We are not treated aggressively for our cancer at first. She, like me, had breast cancer in her past and was in the health care provider's office every six months, begging for help but was told it was arthritis in her shoulder, not the cancer. I told her to try another health care provider. I was told that it was my sickle-cell, but the pain was different. I had found help. The medical health care provider was very helpful, and my friend gave me that tape on supplements that save me. I told Alisha about the supplements, but they were so expensive. Most of the time, we were told it's arthritis, or it's only in your mind and not cancer. There are so many others that are in our situation.—

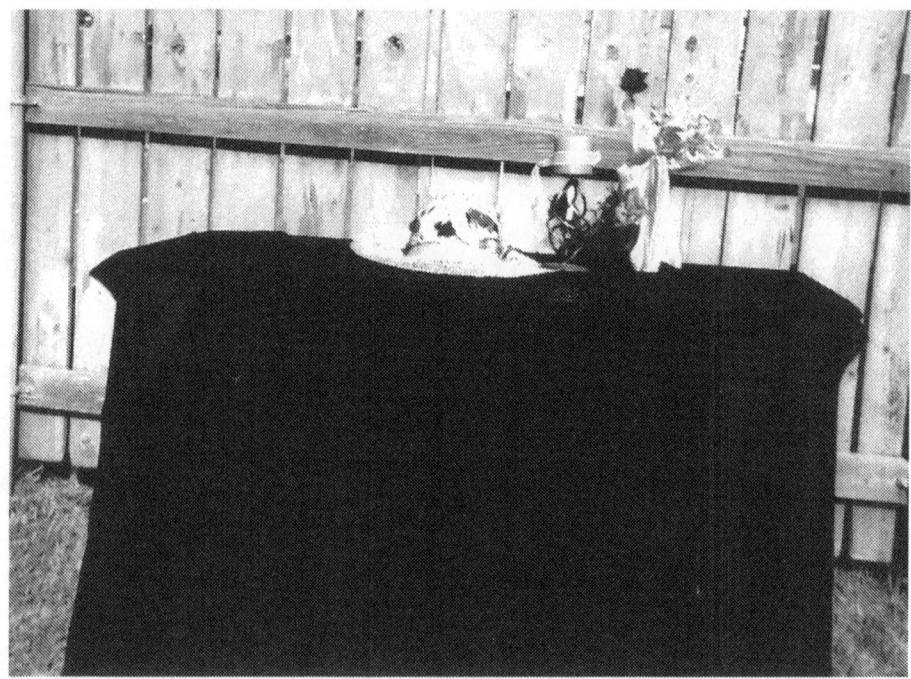

Hello, Diary,

May 18, 2005. I went to my appointment for my Drediv drip, and saw the nurse. She said my MRI test was the same; there were no change in my spine.

Hello, Diary,

June 7, 2005. My stomach and side have been giving me the blues this week. My side is cold; my intestines are not doing their job.

Hello, Diary,

June 21, 2005. I talk to someone at the Quart Clinic about any clinical trials. They did not have anything to fit my needs. So I will move on to the next search; I cannot give up.

Hello, Diary,

June 23, 2005. Today, I went to Glenda to get my monthly treatment. I really need to move closer to my health care provider's office. These seventy miles are getting hard. I need a job, but I am not able to do very much, and I will need to move to a larger city to find a job. This place is too small; there is no help in this town.

Hello, Diary,

June 29, 2005. I am back to Glenda for my CT scan today. The scan did not go well. They did a couple of pictures.

Hello, Diary,

June 30, 2005. A family member had a light stroke, and she is in the hospital. She seems to be okay; her blood pressure is very high. The stroke did not cause any paralysis in any way this time.

Hello, Diary,

July 25, 2005. The health care provider did my colon test today. He said my colon was fine, but I had an infection in my stomach. I will return on August 9, for a follow-up. Maybe he will give me medication for the infection in my stomach.

Hello, Diary,

August 9, 2005. The colon health care provider saw me today. He said I did not need medication for my infection in my stomach, and I would need another colon test in ten years.

Hello, Diary,

August 14, 2005. My friend and I were in a car accident today. We were at the stop light on Grand Avenue. The woman hit us from the back. The crash sounded like the gas tank had blown up. We were taken to the hospital with neck, head, and pain.

Hello, Diary,

August 16, 2005. My head was still hurting this morning since Saturday, so I went to the health care provider today. He gave me some medication for my head.

Hello, Diary,

August 28, 2005. Today, I am in such a bad shape. My body is in pain all over; my flesh is sore and hurting. My skull is sore from the pain on the left side. I have been out of my good vitamins and minerals; they are keeping my immune system fighting the cancer. I have been out of the supplement a couple of weeks, and that car accident did not do my body any good. I am going to have to take some more of my HP this morning.

Hello, Diary,

September 1, 2005. The insurance company sent me a check to fix my car today. It is a shame how that company treated me; they sent me less than half of the estimated damages to fix the car. I cried again at the mistreatment. The estimated amount to fix the car is fourteen hundred dollars, and the lowest is nine hundred dollars. I called a lawyer, which I was trying to avoid doing. His office told me not to cash the check; someone is coming to talk with me tomorrow from their office.

Hello, Diary,

September 16, 2005. I went to Glenda for my cancer treatment, my Drediv drip. I have been dizzy for a couple of days. My blood count must be low again.

Hello, Diary,

September 20, 2005. I went to my local health care provider today for the dizzy spells I am having. He said I have an ear infection that is causing the dizzy spell, so he gave me a prescription.

Hello, Diary,

October 18, 2005. I am tired today. It was back to Glenda, the seventy miles to get my Drediv drip, and to see the health care provider this time. Everything is looking the same, no changes in the treatment. The Drediv, cancer pill, vitamins, and minerals are fighting the cancer back.

Hello, Diary,

October 28, 2005. I am so sick today. My abdomen is infected. I woke up last night at 4:00 a.m. in pain and at the point of vomiting. It's the problem in my left side. There is something that the scans are not picking up in my left abdomen wall and back. Maybe it's tissue that cannot be seen on a CT scan. I am out of my juice, which help my stomach pain. I do not know how I am going to keep getting the vitamins and minerals, because the supplements are so expensive. If I do not take the supplements, my immune system will go back to the condition it was in 2002, and the cancer will soon destroy me; I will die. Your immune system helps fight the cancer. I know a health care provider who treats patients' immune system along with their cancer drugs; it works too. I am in debt. I do not know about the future. I have been saving my empty supplement bottles. They will fill three large garbage bags. I have been treating my immune system since I could not get the help I needed early for this cancer. I have been bleeding and fluid has been leaking in this left side for years, but I could not get a health care provider to listen to me, and help. I am taking some more HP this morning to help with the infection in my side and abdomen.

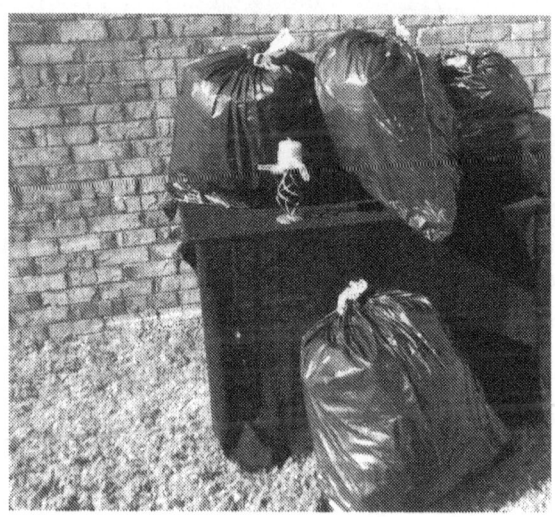

Hello, Diary,

November 14, 2005. I went to get my Drediv drip and the results of my PET scan today. The health care provider said the PET scan picks up some activity around my neck and chest. She is sending me for a CT scan. I am tired; the scans, driving, the seventy miles, and the money. I do not have the money to pay for all of this. I cried on the way home again; it's just getting to be too much. I need a change.


Hello, Diary,

December 6, 2005. I am in pain again; my abdomen and left side. I need someone to look in my abdomen with a scope. Sometimes I feel better than when my other problems start acting up. I do not have any choice but to keep going. I have to do everything for myself, and I am always in pain.


Hello, Diary,

December 12, 2005. Today, when I came from my Drediv treatment, my body was stinging all over. I had to go to bed. All last night, this tumor in my side was bubbling and leaking in my system. I have been out of my vitamins and minerals for a week now, but I order some, and they should arrive this week. My body is sore all over; it is as if my system is being poisoned. When I try to go without my vitamins and minerals, the cancer starts taking over my body. My only chance is to keep treating my own immune system.


Hello, Diary,

January 10, 2006. Today, my bones are really hurting and stinging. My Drediv is out of my system, and I am out of some of my supplements. I will get my Drediv drip; soon, this will help me. I am in trouble health wise and financially too. I do not know what I am going to do. I need a job, but both of my hands are hurting and sore. Where can I find employment in this shape? It will be hard to do most work on schedules.

Hello, Diary,

January 11, 2006. This morning, my brother Earl called to tell me that my friend's brother has died. I have been sick myself this week. I will try to go to see her family. I will get a friend to go with me.


Hello, Diary,

January 12, 2006. Gean, Dean, and I went to my friend's mother's home to give our condolence to the family. All three of us knew someone in that family. My friend and I graduated from high school together. When she heard that my cancer had come back; she came to my aid. On the way home, I thought how this could be me dead. I have been in so much pain lately, and my family could be needing condolence. Life is so fragile. It seems that you are doing fine, but you can really be suffering. My friend looked the picture of health.


Hello, Diary,

January 12, 2006. Today, everything is infected: my eyes, down my leg, even under my feet is stinging and itching from this infection leaking into my system from the left side of my abdomen. I will take some more of the HP.


Hello, Diary,

January 16, 2006. I had to see a local health care provider. My body is so infected that it is coming out of my eyes; they are itching and stinging too, from my stomach down my left foot and toes. The health care provider said I have a urinary tract infection and eye infection, so he gave me two prescriptions.


Hello, Diary,

January 18, 2006. Today, my stomach is still feeling infected. I have been taking the pill for three days now. My eyes are somewhat better. Could the infection is a result of the cancer?

Hello, Diary,

January 30, 2006. I had to go to the emergency room for my eyes and stomach. They are still infected. The health care provider did a kidney x-ray and an EKG. I told him what prescriptions the health care provider had given me a few weeks ago, so this health care provider gave me two shots and another prescription. My eyes are stinging all around the eye socket and eye lids. He said they were red and parched; my skin is dried out on top of my eye lids from the infection coming out of them.

Hello, Diary,

February 6, 2006. I drove to Glenda to get my Drediv drip today. I am so tired. The seventy miles there and seventy back my body is exhausted. When I made it home, I receive a call telling me that Earl was in the hospital, so I have to drive another forty miles and back before I go to bed today. God, please help us.

Hello, Diary,

February 9, 2006. Today has been a sad and painful day for our family. Our brother, Earl, died today. This is the second brother we have lost in death. It's like a piece of me is dying every time one of them dies. Death is truly an enemy to the human race. He was in a car accident in 1998. He has been sick the last few months; we did not know it was that serious. I saw his suffering last night. He was in so much pain. He couldn't catch his breath because of the spasms due to his being paralyzed. I had the opportunity to stay the night with him, and I saw the pain he has been suffering at home when he had spasms like these. He went to sleep about three o'clock this morning. I thought the worse of the trouble was over with for him. This morning we talked, and the health care provider was going to let him go home today. He ate his breakfast, but in less than an hour, he was dead. It is hard for our family seeing another brother die this soon. He is a unique brother. We will miss him very much. He was always ready to help. A car accident left him completely paralyzed for the last eight years. He was only forty-six last month. My other brother was thirty-one when he died ten years ago. It's really going to be hard with both of them dead.

Hello, Diary,

February 11, 2006. There are so many things to do for the funeral, and this eye infection has returned this week. The pills cleared it up some last week, but it's back. I may have to see an eye specialist.


Hello, Diary,

February 14, 2006. Our brother's funeral was today. We are so sad, and it was a great loss. He was so kind to all of us. Even though he was the one who needed the most in the last eight years, he gave so much to everyone. Family, friends, and the community all came to our aid today. It was such a great blessing to receive their help at time of sorrow. Thanks.


Hello, Diary,

February 15, 2006. It's the day after the funeral, and all five of us are tired and sick: me, my two sisters, and my sister's two children. Today, we are at the trial for the car accident we had in 2004. The person in the other car parked in the highway. Her lawyer was great in her case. Even though we were hurt, she told the jury that we did not seek much medical help. We were lying together. I have twelve health care provider visits on my medical insurance a year; and I have two major health problems and cannot afford to go to the health care provider when I need treatment for them. So when I took the brace off my fractured arm after I felt it was healed and did not make another medical bill that I could not afford, her lawyer said I was not hurt. My sister and I have so many medical bills that we cannot pay now, and her lawyer did just what we knew they would, give us nothing for our injury. She and the jury put all the blame on my nephew, who was driving our car. We are still hurting in every way. It's over with, and we can go and try to live.


Hello, Diary,

March 6, 2006. I receive my Drediv drip today. My blood was low as usual. My body has been in severe pain the past few weeks, but I feel better today. The pain is always in my abdomen.

Hello, Diary,

March 7, 2006. I was going to my family health care provider today because of the pain in my stomach, but when I heard on the news that Mrs. Joe had died, I thought what's the use, I will just keep living as long I can like this, pain and all. Nothing will help; just keep taking my vitamins and minerals.

Hello, Diary,

March 16, 2006. I am in pain tonight. I did a lot of running around taking care of business for myself and others today. I do not have anyone to do my business. Sometimes I have to do lots of running for others too. My heart is flatting, my abdomen, back, and legs are stinging; the cancer has spread all over my body. I double up my vitamins and minerals this week, maybe this will help my body's immune system to fight the cancer.

Hello, Diary,

March 25, 2006. Today, my body is sore from my waist down even the muscles and bones, and both my legs are sore. It was like this yesterday; it is even worse today. I am pushing on as normal. If I stop, I will die. I am trying to keep going as long as I can. Everyone is sick, so there is no reason to talk about my problem. Sometimes it's like my body is probably closing down. I am going out in my volunteer work. This way I will be with people. It will take my mind off the problem and pain.

Hello, Diary,

April 1, 2006. I have felt better today than I have in weeks. My blood has been really low, but I have been working hard to get the blood count up. I double up all my vitamins, minerals, and juice. I bought some beta-carotene and took them. My flesh and bones have been hurting and sore for weeks. I am in debt over my head, but it's debt or death for me. I want to live too.

Hello, Diary,

April 3, 2006. Today, I went to get my Drediv drip. My blood was seven and twenty-three which is normal for me. I have some swelling in the lymph nodes. My throat has been sore this week.

Hello, Diary,

April 27, 2006. This morning, my back is hurting; my kidney is infected on both sides of my body. My stomach is swollen and stinging. My whole body is in pain; I am sick as a wet dog. Any time I do any walking, the cancer flares up all over my body. I feel like my belly should be opened and my organs should be removed, but what would be left? This has been going on too long. Thanks for my cancer treatments and the supplement, all the vitamins and minerals that I am taking to fight the cancer. I am still alive.

Hello, Diary,

May 3, 2006. Today was Drediv drip day. The nurse said my blood count was up a point to twenty-four, which was good because I worked hard to get it up. My kidney is infected. I have had to take my H P today. I feel that deep stinging on the side of my head, the skull is sore too.

Hello, Diary,

May 10, 2006. The nurse from my health care provider's office called today to say that the health care provider will be cutting back on my Drediv to every three months; that my scans look good, yet the scans don't tell what is happening to the cancer in my flesh. I am taking all of these vitamins, mineral, and everything else that I cannot afford to stay alive. My whole body is getting worse; the cancer has affected all of my organs in my abdomen. My kidneys are infected. All the tests say I am doing good. If the test could feel what I feel.

Hello, Diary,

May 13, 2006. My best friend gave me some more vitamins. I thank her because I am a day or two from being completely out of supplements. I am thankful for a friend like her.

Hello, Diary,

May 16, 2006. My back has been hurting for a week on both sides now; one side has hurt off and on for years. I have an appointment with the urologist on May 30. Most likely the same nodes will be on my kidney that has been hurting for years. The tumor should have been removed years ago.

Hello, Diary,

May 30, 2006. I saw the urologist today. He ordered a CT scan on my kidney. He will call me when he gets the result of the scans.

Hello, Diary,

June 2, 2006. I receive the results of the kidney scan from the urologist today. He said I have the same lesion on my kidney; they have not gotten any larger than last year. They have been there for years. Are they are cancerous now?

Hello, Diary,

June 13, 2006. This is the second time I have experienced what the health care provider asked me about when she told me the cancer was on my spine back in 2002. I am frighten, because something must be going wrong with my spine and my whole body. It's only because I keep treating my immune system to fight that I am not experiencing the full results of the cancer. When I try to go without my supplement for some time, I start experiencing in my spine what the health care provider said I would experience. I have been taking the vitamins and minerals faithfully for four years, twice a day and some time three times a day. They have help my body to fight back the full effects of the cancer.

Hello, Diary,

June 14, 2006. I am trying to hold out the three months without getting my Drediv drip. My body is in such bad condition from the cancer. I cannot stay off the Drediv for the full three months. I am concern about how low in my vitamins and minerals. I do not know how much longer I will be able to continue with the vitamins and minerals; they are one of the things keeping me alive. If I stop taking the vitamins, I will not be able to get out of bed or walk, because the pain is so bad in my back and body. I have increased my vitamins this month, but I have still been able to feel the stinging in my bones and flesh. I have called every organization I thought could help me, but no one would help me. I need a job, but who in this place is going to hire me with my medical record? I just do not know what to do anymore. I want to live too, as long as I can, so where do I go next?

Hello, Diary,

June 18, 2006. I did some walking this weekend. I had My yearly meeting for three days. The last two days, my whole body is sore and swollen. It will take a couple of days of bed rest to get my body back in shape. Days like these let me know that the cancer is still affecting my whole body. Most of the time, the pain is from my waist down my legs. Now my internal organs are affected from the little walking I did on Saturday and Sunday. There was a floor full of sick people at our meeting; more people are sick than ever before. We need a change badly, and soon.

Hello, Diary,

June 20, 2006.

June 20, 2006, I receive some more of my good vitamins, so I will take these to try to help my body to fight. The stinging in my stomach is causing it to swell sometime. The test says everything is the same every time they come back, but my body is saying something different. I am dying! I need the finance to keep up the high-price supplement program that I am on that is keeping me alive. I have searched high and low and have not been able to find anyone who can help financially with the supplement. That is why I want to start a nonprofit program for cancer patients.

Hello, Diary,

June 26, 2006. I have been doubling my supplements, and decided to call my health care provider to see if they can start giving my Drediv drip again. They gave me an appointment for July 1. I had to do some walking last week, and everything hurts, back, legs, feet, and even my stomach is swollen. The insurance needs to pay for supplements for cancer patients too. The vitamins and minerals help the patients to build immune system to fight cancer.

Hello, Diary,

July 1, 2006. I receive my Drediv drip today; maybe my bones will feel better in a few days. My blood count was back at twenty-three; last time I had gotten it up to twenty-four. I ran out my good vitamins and minerals in May. I am going to try to get the count back up. Thankful, they made the adjustment for me.

Hello, Diary,

July 5, 2006. My organs are sore. I had to take some HP. My flesh is sore, and it is hard for me to walk today, with my legs and feet in pain.

Hello, Diary,

July 13, 2006. I have been limping all this week because of the pain in my feet. My blood is not circulating through my system and reaching my feet. I can get the health care provider will give me something for arthritis, but it could be the cancer in my abdomen that is causing problems in my circulatory system.

Hello, Diary,

July 15, 2006. I have a PET scan next Tuesday, and it's in a city about 160 miles away. I don't have any idea of how I will get there. I will have to take myself, sick and all, in my old car.

Hello, Diary,

July 16, 2006. Today, I am going to get me some more of the supplement that I have been on since 2002, to add to what I am taking. The nerve in my spine is flaring up again badly, my leg and feet numb. I am in serious trouble in every way; something needs to change soon for me. I called my health care provider's office to find out if my insurance will pay for the PET scan next week. They say it will; that's why they are sending me to Ford. Financially, I cannot pay $3,700 for the test. I will have to credit the $50 for the gas. I need to be closer to my treatment center.

Hello, Diary,

July 18, 2006. Today, I had to drive myself the almost 160 miles to Ford for my PET scan. A friend went with me in my little beat-up car. When I made it to the testing center, they told me that all testing had been rescheduled for the twentieth. I was so hurt; I do not have the money to come back on the twentieth. So I will try to get my health care provider to make another appointment later. I used money I did not have for this trip. I am sick, and I had to drive these 160 miles to no avail.

Hello, Diary,

July 24, 2006. I called my health care provider's office and ask them to change my appointment with the heath care provider from August to September because I did not get the PET scan yet. I will have to make another appointment in September to see the health care provider. They gave me an appointment for my Dredia drip on August 10, 2006.

Hello, Diary,

July 31, 2006. Today, my friend and I are going to ride to Nashville with my sister. She is moving to Nashville this week to be near her children. So we will stay until Sunday, and take the bus home.

Hello, Diary,

August 6, 2006. We had a nice time in Nashville last week. My health held up. I did not do much walking. Some friends invited us over to their home, and one mother and daughter took us by car to see the city of Nashville and to dinner. That was fun; we thank them for the tour of the city. It is nice to be able to enjoy good friends in new places. They were new in the town, but she gave us a nice car tour of the city. I cannot walk to see the sights anymore, so I would have stayed at home if those girls had opened their home and time to me. My body is affected sometimes from the waist down by walking.

Hello, Diary,

August 9, 2006. I am feeling so bad this morning. Last night I was dizzy, the room spinning when I turn over in the bed. Again as the last time, I went to the local health care provider, and he gave me a prescription for ear infection, but could this have something to do with the cancer on my skull. It is always on the left side of my head. It makes me vomit from the spinning. I have to get up and sit up. After sitting up the rest of the night, I feel better, but I am weak, so I will increase my vitamins and minerals to boost my immune system to keep fighting the cancer.

Hello, Diary,

August 10, 2006. I receive my Drediv drip today. I am tired from the long drive. My blood count has dropped again. I feel washed out. My PET scan is on August 18, 2006, so I will get an appointment to see the health care provider sometime in September. This body is wearing out. Everything is stinging and sore today. HELP.

Hello, Diary,

August 19, 2006. I went to get my PET scan in Ford yesterday. I was sick but I had to drive the hundred and sixty miles there and back. My sister went with me, but she is sick too. The testing center is going to send my results to my health care provider's office. They will send the CT scan back to the hospital too.

Hello, Diary,

August 26, 2006. I had to go and get some calcium today from Blackstone. My friend drove me to pick up the calcium. If I don't have it, I just cannot move; my bones are in so much pain. I am out of my good vitamins, so I am hurting. I do not have the money to get them, and my cards are maxed out. So I do not know what I am going to do for next month's supply. My body will start going down sooner than it is now. The supplement is helping my body to fight the cancer. I know there are thousands of women in my situation who need help with no one to turn to for the help, poor, needy, and all along.

Hello, Diary,

August 29, 2006. I have been thinking about asking an official of the city if they have grant money to help develop programs for the citizens of the city. So today, I push myself to go and talk to the official about the matter. I ask him if the city could provide me with some grant money and a building to start a vitamin and mineral program for breast cancer patients and others. He, said the city did not have any grants or building they could offer me. He told me about two people whom I could try to talk to about the program that I want to start.

Hello, Diary,

September 1, 2006. I contacted the persons that the official told me about, and I have an appointment with one on Thursday, September 7.

Hello, Diary,

September 4, 2006. The body is talking to me today. I do not have any of my good vitamins, and it is time for my Drediv drip which helps my bones and keep the stinging under control. I will call to order some as soon as I can. I am going to try to get out of the house at eleven o'clock with my friend, so I will not be home crying all day. I am taking the cheap vitamins that I have on hand, but they do not fight the cancer like the potent vitamins.

Hello, Diary,

September 13, 2006. I tried to contact one of the persons who are getting together a nonprofit program there in town soon. I had talked with him last month. He said there was a group of women who were cancer patients that was looking to start a program to help cancer patients. He is out of town, working on getting his program up and running.

Hello, Diary,

September 19, 2006. Today, I turned in an application for a substitute teacher position in a county school. I need some extra finance to continue getting my immune-strengthening supplements. I also spoke with the person that is put to gather the nonprofit program. He said he would pass my name and telephone onto the group of other women that are trying to get a program established in town. I also asked the other official to give a letter to an official of the state. Who, I think can help us in the future with our program. If I die sooner than later, it is not because I have not asked for help, I surely have looked under every ROCK. One day there will be a "yes, I will help you." I shall keep trying until I am unable to.

Hello, Diary,

September 21, 2006. It is about six o'clock. I feel like I am dying; my whole body is stinging, my head, eyes, ribs, arms, fingers, stomach, intestines, spine, legs, and even my toes are stinging. It has been almost two months since I could afford my immune-building vitamins. I feel like my body is closing down if I do not get my good vitamins soon. My body is swollen every morning I awake now. When I sit in a certain position in a chair or on a couch, it really affects my spine and my whole body. This started back in 2000 when I first noticed that I was having difficulty in walking and sitting. It had gotten progressively worse over the years. I have a special chair that I use for long-term sitting at home, and out I have to be careful to where I sit, but sometimes I do not have a choice, like today, and that is the reason I am crying now in pain. As I lay across my bed in pain crying, a friend calls to say hello. We met at a hospital in her town when I went for my PET scan, so she asked how I was doing. I told her that I was being treated for breast cancer, and I was in her town to get some test. She said she knows a person who is using herbs to fight her cancer, and she is doing well. So, she is going to call me on the weekend with her telephone number, Standing for Cancer! I crawled back to bed, no longer crying. How thankful I am for friends.


Hello, Diary,

October 3, 2006. Back to Glenda for my treatment today. The body is stinging; I drove, but my sister went with me. I receive my Drediv drip. I also receive my PET scan results. They showed some arthritis at the base of my neck and in my lower back. The health care provider said things look good. The blood count stays low. The cancer drugs and my six thousand dollars of vitamins and minerals over the past three years are keeping me alive. If there were only a test that could tell how really you are feeling today. I have not had my expensive vitamins and minerals for two months; by the test, I should be feeling, great. I order the supplements last week, so I should get them this week. I will keep treating my immune system to help fight the cancer as long as I can financially. I cannot give up yet.


Hello, Diary,

November 1, 2006. My sister and I went to Glenda to get my Drediv drip. I feel okay today. My vitamins are back in my system. I look around in some of the stores in the town. I found me a nice little hat, and put it on there since it was cool today. We also shopped for groceries, ate, and headed for home. It was a good day. My blood count is back at seven and twenty-three, but it stays low.


Hello, Diary,

November 2006. We had the funeral of a friend today who had cancer and who was two years older than I am. It makes me gnash my teeth when I see all of my young family and friends dying like this. What's wrong? I know I would be dead too if my friend had not given me that tape on vitamins and minerals to strengthen the immune system. My body was going down fast back then, and there was no help to be had, everyone was saying I was fine, the test came back fine too. In 2002 the test my health care provider ran did not came back not fine, and that gave me a push to do something. My best friend remembers the tape she had listened to in the past talking about the immune system and cancer, she gave it to me to listen. It made sense; I started doing what it said on the tape while I looked for medical help. When we are diagnosed with diseases, we need to try to educate yourself as much as we can on the cause and treatment of our disease, so we can live a little longer.

Hello, Diary,

November 12, 2006. Today is a bad day for me. I need some of my juice for my stomach, and my abdomen is really infected. I am going to get some soon; I have been off the juice for almost three months now. The stomach and everything else in my abdomen is in pain today. I just must keep going because if I stop, I think I will give up the fight to stay alive. So with the help of the Almighty, I keep on moving.

Hello, Diary,

November 14, 2006. My body has been so infected the last few days I had to go to the local health care provider. My eyes are infected. I just feel so bad all over my body. The health care provider gave me a prescription for the infection. I am still building my immune system with my vitamins and minerals to fight the cancer. Some times it seems the cancer is winning the fight, like this week. It is a hard fight, physically, emotionally, and financially. I do not want to give up the fight against the cancer.

Hello, Diary,

November 21, 2006. I am feeling much better today. I think my infection has cleared up. I am still looking at organizations that I think may help me to get a program started to help patients with cancer to get vitamins and minerals to build their immune system to fight the cancer. This has helped me to keep alive so far.

Hello, Diary,

November 28, 2006. My Drediv is out of my system; the bones are stinging more today. I will get it again on December 4, next week. I am experiencing nerve pain from my neck down my shoulders and arms too. I have not been able to afford my good vitamins lately. So I can feel some of the effects of not being on them for sometime.

Hello, Diary,

December 3, 2006. Tomorrow, I will go to Glenda to get my Drediv drip, which will help the bones to feel better. Tuesday, my best bud is having back surgery, so I want to go, to be there with her. The next two days, I am going to need lots of H.S. for strength. My left side is acting up today. I am taking everything I have, but I am out of some supplements.

Hello, Diary,

December 13, 2006. The left side of my head, behind my eye and face, is hurting this week. I do not usually have headaches. It is just on the left side of my head. The nerves in my neck are still tightened up; really, I have been feeling so bad lately. I really need a CT scan on my head and neck soon. My vitamins and minerals have helped to build my immune system to fight the cancer so far. I am still trying to stay on the supplement. My shipment of vitamins came today at a great expense.

Hello, Diary,

December 30, 2006. My body is aching and stinging more lately, my Dradiv is out of my system. My bones start to feel weak and sting. I have another week before I get my treatment. The Dradiv does work at keeping the bones stronger. I am thankful that my health care provider put me on this drug, and it has worked so good for me. I still have some of my expensive supplements, so I hope they will help me to go through next week until I get my Dradiv.

Hello, Diary,

January 8, 2007. I receive my Dradiv and I have been feeling dizzy and my flesh is stinging. I am just feeling bad. The pain is always there in my abdomen; it's all over, my insides is infected. I asked the nurse to send me to get a CT scan of my head and chest.

Hello, Diary,

January 28, 2007. Today, my ears are ringing, my head is spinning when I turn it or move in a certain way. My friends do not know that I was about to pass out. I was praying, "Please, God, do not let me pass out." My head has been getting dizzy lately. I do not know why. I did not have high blood pressure. What is going on in my body?

## Object

To Establish a Vitamine and Mineral Program for Cancer Patients

## Acknowledgement

To God, Family, Friends and ALL my medical teams, who has helped me make this journey, Thanks.

www.ingramcontent.com/pod-product-compliance
Lightning Source LLC
Chambersburg PA
CBHW021303280526
45784CB00005B/2497